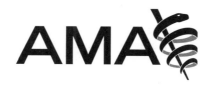

D0986671

WHAT TO DO BEFORE, DURING, AND AFTER AN EMERGENCY OR DISASTER:

A Preparedness Toolkit for Office-based Health Care Practices

Kristine M. Gebbie, DrPH, RN
Joan Grabe Dean (acting)
School of Nursing, Hunter College
City University of New York
New York, New York

James James, MD, DrPH, MHA
Editor-in-Chief, *Disaster Medicine and Public Health Preparedness*
Director, Center for Public Health Preparedness and Disaster Response
American Medical Association
Chicago, Illinois

Italo Subbarao, DO, MBA
Deputy Editor, *Disaster Medicine and Public Health Preparedness*
Director of the Public Health Readiness Office,
Center for Public Health Preparedness and Disaster Response
American Medical Association
Chicago, Illinois

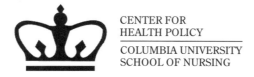

CENTER FOR
HEALTH POLICY

COLUMBIA UNIVERSITY
SCHOOL OF NURSING

Prepared by the AMA Public Health Readiness Office and
Columbia University School of Nursing Center for Health Policy

Cover photo credits: Left to right, row by row, from top, Brand X, Sean Locke/istockphoto.com, FhotoDisc, Creatas, Jupiter Images, Jupiter Images, and Jupiter Images; Background: PhotoDisc.

Internet address: www.ama-assn.org

Additional copies of this book may be ordered by calling 800 621-8335 or from the secure AMA Web site at www.amabookstore.com.
Refer to product number OP323709.

ISBN 978-1-60359-202-4
BP01:OP323709:05/09

ABOUT THIS TOOLKIT

Chicken Little shouting "the sky is falling" is balanced by the just-in-time television anthem of "here comes the Cavalry." Indeed, these represent two extremes of the disaster preparedness spectrum that are neither realistic nor even desirable.

As clinicians, we are prepared to deal with individual patient emergencies, and courses such as CPR, ACLS and PALS are well known educational tools. These tools provide us with the knowledge and opportunity to practice in a controlled environment so during times of an individual patient crisis, when seconds count, we are prepared.

Like individual patient emergencies, community disasters are going to happen, sometime. This toolkit serves as the foundation to construct your Office Emergency Preparedness Plan.

Objectives
This toolkit will help you:
1. assess your practice and community vulnerability
2. determine what is needed to maintain your business' continuity
3. create an emergency preparedness plan for your practice
4. train your staff to the plan and evaluate the staff's readiness through participation in drill and exercises
5. connect with local emergency management planners to better understand how your resources and expertise can be used during an emergency response.

Whether you are the lead clinician, the office manager or administrator, this tool is for you.

The toolkit provides an outline of steps to be taken and includes forms and tables as templates. Emphasis is on connecting with local partners in order for the office-based practice to become part of the local planning process and tailor your plan to match local expectation.

The toolkit was developed through a two-day workshop sponsored by

Columbia University and the American Medical Association. The working group participants included Kristine Gebbie, DrPH, RN; Jacqueline Merrill, DrNSc, MPH, RN; James James, MD, DrPH, MHA; Italo Subbarao, DO, MBA; Joseph C. Dreyfus, MD; Darrel E. Lovins, DO, MPH, FACOFP; John A. Mitas, MD, FACP; Raymond Swienton, MD, FACEP; David T. Hannan, MD, MPA; Gerald E. Harmon, MD, FAAFP. Comments have been solicited and received from the interdisciplinary board of the National Disaster Life Support Educational Foundation, and reviewers included physicians, nurses, dentists, and healthcare system emergency managers.

This document is a component of a National Training Strategy for medical providers, a collaborative effort of the New York Consortium for Emergency Preparedness Continuing Education. Funding is from the Office of the Assistant Secretary for Preparedness and Response, Department of Health and Human Services (T01 HP01411). It is neither a professional standard nor a legal document, but a useful tool to assist your practice in developing a custom plan to serve your community's needs.

We would like to thank the following authors and organizations for granting reprint permission: Dr. Scott Needle and the Mississippi Chapter of the American Academy of Pediatrics, author and publisher respectively of *A Disaster Preparedness Plan for Pediatricians* (2006); Cliff Rapp, licensed healthcare risk manager and Vice President of Risk Management at First Professionals Insurance Company, Inc. (FPIC), is the author of *Disaster and Recovery Plan: Physician Office Practice* (2005)[1]; and the Kentucky Medical Association for *Model Disaster Plan for a Physician Practice*.

[1] FPIC is a leading professional liability insurer. Mr. Rapp is widely published and an international speaker on loss prevention and risk management.

CONTENTS

If disaster struck today, what would happen at your office? Would your patients know what to do, how to reach you for medications or their patient records? Do you have contingencies in place to continue caring for your patients? Would your staff know what to do? Could you assist in a community-wide emergency response?

If our answer to any (or all) of these questions is "no," and changing them to "yes" seems overwhelming, help is in your hands. Through the steps contained in this toolkit, you will learn how to minimize the impacts of an emergency, improving not only your ability to continue delivery of clinical services during the emergency, but also to restore your practice to normalcy more quickly and efficiently.

This toolkit contains planning tools to help you predict the need for essential supplies, staff assistance, local resources, and appropriate sources for financial assistance. It will help you assess the likely hazards your community faces, identify the challenges you may encounter both during an emergency and after, and define the roles and responsibilities vital to clear communication, a key to surviving disasters large and small.

Still overwhelmed? Know that you are not in this alone; a national effort is underway to increase local preparedness. Your

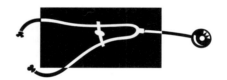

Practices Large and Small
Does Size Matter?

According to the American College of Physicians, 48% of Internists (including Internal Medicine sub-specialists) work in "small practices," i.e., comprising fewer than five physicians.

According to the American Dental Association, 83% of dentists work in "small practices," comprising two or fewer dentists. Of these, 63% are working in solo practices.

If your practice is small, look for the "Small Practice Tips," which will help you custom fit certain planning steps to your size.

local emergency management agency, local health department, local hospital(s), the American Medical Association (AMA), the American Dental Association (ADA), and many other professional associations have already begun their plans and can serve as valuable resources while you develop yours.

By creating an emergency response plan for your office-based practice, you are not only ensuring the best possible recovery of your practice in the wake of an emergency—you are demonstrating the highest possible level of commitment to your staff, your patients, and your community, that you (and your practice) will be there when they need you most.

Setting the Stage: Your Role in an Emergency

Figure 1 illustrates how the clinician, the office-based practice, and the community are linked in the emergency preparedness process.

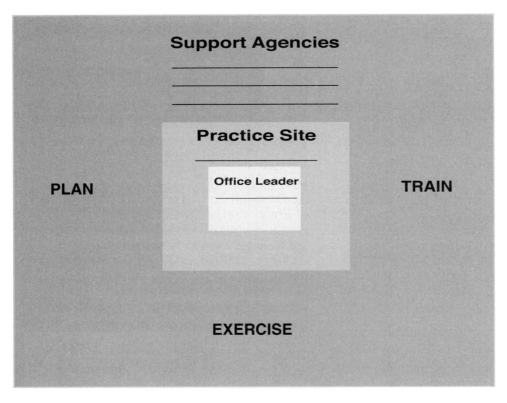

Emergency Preparedness Model

FIGURE 1
The Emergency Preparedness Model

You and Your Office

At the center is the individual responsible for the office-based practice—i.e., the physician, physician assistant, nurse practitioner, dentist, chiropractor, veterinarian or office manager. By adequately preparing yourself and your office staff for the personal impact of an emergency, your practice will have a better chance of staying open during an emergency and/or of recovering from the crisis. (See **Appendix A** for the **Emergency Contact Card**, **Family Emergency Plan** and **Emergency Preparedness Medical Needs Checklist (for patients)** templates).

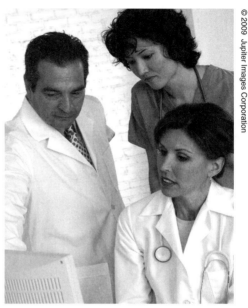

© 2009 Jupiter Images Corporation

Your Office and the Community

Your practice also has a role to play during emergencies—to provide for and communicate with your patient population within the community (see box on page 4 for potential roles your practice can fill in your community).

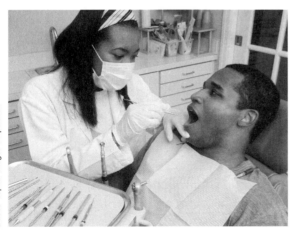

© 2009 Jupiter Images Corporation

Your office's effectiveness will depend on whether you have a plan for contingency operations and a staff prepared to carry it out. During a crisis, the success of the health care community response system relies on the readiness of office-based practices and the individuals who work there. Optimally, success will require communication and cooperation from other health care and non-health care partners; all parties need to share and compare plans beforehand to know how to engage with one another during an emergency. Once you understand the expectations of your community, you will need to balance them against the economic realities of your practice in order to determine the level of investment you are able to make in emergency preparedness. **For more about the potential costs of emergency preparedness, see Appendix D.**

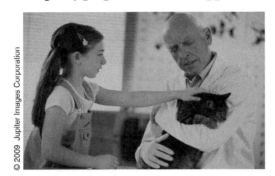

© 2009 Jupiter Images Corporation

Your affiliation with the local health department and/or local hospital is an asset to the community. Maintaining a dialogue about emergency preparedness with these partners is an essential role you can play. These linkages will create communication channels

How Will You Respond to an Emergency?

Here are some examples:

- Keep your practice open to triage your own patients; use your answering machine or Web site to share emergency messages in coordination with the local office of emergency management and as part of the overall community response plan (e.g., during a major weather event).

- Keep your practice open to accept referrals for patients as directed by your community's response plan (e.g., serve as secondary triage or overflow site for the local hospital emergency department (ED) to provide care for the "minimally" injured or affected).

- Close your practice to care and send staff elsewhere for duty as directed by your community's response plan (e.g., they serve as added or "surge" staff for a

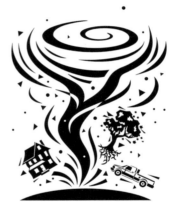

© 2009 Jupiter Images Corporation

hospital or at a shelter needing medical personnel).

- Close your practice completely, directing both scheduled and emergency patients to other sites for care via instructions left on your practice answering machine, with an answering service, or via another mechanism.

This toolkit will enable you to create a plan like one of these scenarios adapted to your unique circumstances.

In Case of Emergency, Can You Reach These VIPs?

- Mayor or county executive
- Fire department
- Police department
- Emergency medical services
- Public works department
- Telephone company
- Electric and gas utilities
- Insurance agent
- Banker

- The American Red Cross
- Local houses of worship
- Internet service provider
- Pharmacies
- Real estate agent (if relocation is needed)
- Electronic medical record (EMR) data warehouse or technical support
- Medical supplier
- Alarm company

through which, for example, you will be able to continue to provide medical care to your most vulnerable patient population, provide accurate information to all of your patients, and inform the local incident emergency management team about your capabilities. If you do not already have a relationship with your health department, for example, now would be a good time to start.

There are multiple agencies and groups that have a role in emergency planning and response. You may find yourself working with local businesses and other organizations, including those listed above. Your plan should include collecting contact information for the key people at these organizations in your community.

In A Hurry?

✓ If you prefer to skip the whys and hows one needs to plan and get right to it, we have provided "Skimmer Boxes" throughout the narrative of this toolkit to direct the reader to the pertinent form(s) in the Appendices for that particular step.

Emergency Planning Cycle for Office-based Health Care Practices

Planning for emergencies can be described as a cycle of critical steps. The figure below describes these steps, which are needed for creating and maintaining an emergency response plan for your office-based practice. Ideally, this cycle should be completed at least annually.

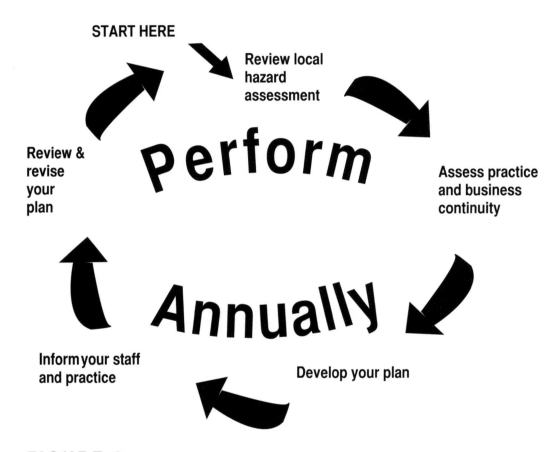

FIGURE 2
The Emergency Planning Cycle

The Essential Components of a Complete Disaster (Emergency) Response

1. **Personal and Family Preparedness.** The Family Emergency Plan by Ready.gov and the Emergency Contact Card by the American Red Cross are provided for you and your staff to complete. **The Emergency Preparedness Medical Needs Checklist** can be distributed by you to assist patients in planning for uninterrupted medical care during emergencies. Templates are provided in **Appendix A.**

2. **Office Practices/Patients.** Following the steps in this tool-kit will result in a plan that will prepare you for contingencies so you can continue providing care to your patients during a disaster.

3. **Community.** Contact local health or emergency response agencies to become connected to these plans. Ways to become more involved in local emergency response efforts are listed in **Appendix B.**

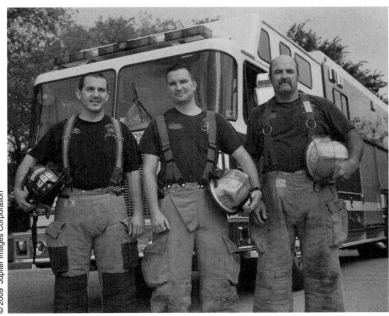

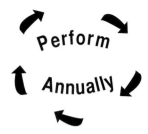

Perform Annually

STEP 1.
REVIEW THE LOCAL
HAZARD ASSESSMENT

There is a difference between a **risk** and a **hazard**. A *hazard* is anything that has the potential to do harm to property, the environment, and/or people. *Risk* is the probability of that hazard potential actually occurring. You need to be aware of and consider both as you develop your plan.

Hazards vary from community to community. Climate and earthquake zones, proximity to the seacoast or a major river, and local industrial or transportation activity can affect the likelihood of an event causing an emergency. Identify the more likely hazards in your area based on local risk factors and take them into account in developing your plan.

Types of hazards include (but are not limited to):

- Natural, human-made, or technological disasters (e.g., snowstorms, terrorism, a blackout)
- Accidental and intentional events (e.g., a burst pipe, a shooter on a rampage)
- Internal and external events (e.g., a fire, a flood)
- Controllable events and those beyond an organization's control (e.g., undiagnosed persons, a flu pandemic)
- Events with prior warning and those without (e.g., hurricanes vs. most earthquakes).

As part of a national effort to improve their emergency response preparedness, your local or state emergency management agency, local health department, or local hospital have also considered these risks and may have a local hazard assessment or vulnerability analysis they would willingly share with you. Although you may need to make small adjustments to their assessment based on the specifics of your site and past experience, starting with their assessment will simplify and speed up your work.

Whether adapting an available analysis or developing your own, the following example of a local hazard assessment (see Table 1 on page 10) will help you complete your own. A clean template is provided in **Appendix C**.

Table 1. Hazard Vulnerability Analysis for Community Practice Sites

To calculate your health center's vulnerability to hazards, enter the appropriate number in each box (on page 11)and total for that hazard. We have listed several in each category that are of concern; you may want to add one or more hazards, or describe one of the hazards in more detail, because of your particular local concerns. The higher the point total, the greater the overall impact of the event on the practice site.

"Probability" = the frequency at which the hazardous event occurs.

  5 points: Happens annually

  4 points: Has happened within the past 2–5 years

  3 points: Has happened within the past 5–10 years

  2 points: Has happened over 10 years ago

  1 point: Has never happened before

"Overall Impact on Center" = the impact that the particular hazard has caused (or could cause) in the way of physical damage to the center, staffing shortages, interruption of patient services, and/or supply disruption.

  5 points: Severe impact on center (has caused center to close)

  4 points: Significant impact on center

  3 points: Moderate impact on center

  2 points: Minimal impact on center

  1 point: No impact on center

"Overall Impact on Community" = on average, the impact that the particular hazard has caused overall to the wider community in the past.

  5 points: Has required a federal response

  4 points: Has required a state government response

  3 points: Has required a county government response

  2 points: Has been resolved with a local response

  1 point: No response necessary

EXAMPLE:

HAZARDS	PROBABILITY	OVERALL IMPACT ON CENTER	OVERALL IMPACT ON COMMUNITY	TOTAL
Natural Hazards				
Flood	5	3	3	11
Earthquake	1	1	1	3
Tornado	3	5	4	12
Industrial Hazards				
Fire	2	5	2	9
Blackout	4	4	3	11

In this instance, the likelihood of a flood occurring is greater than a tornado. Although the impact of the tornado on the center would be high, it is advisable to spend more time or energy preparing for an event that happens annually, as compared to one that happens less frequently. You should be certain to include in your plan contingencies for any hazard that scores **10 or higher.** This is not to say that those hazards that fall below 10 points should not be planned for, but rather that greater emphasis should be placed on the more frequently occurring, higher impact hazards.

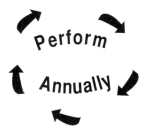

Perform Annually

STEP 2.
ASSESSSING
HEALTH CARE
PRACTICE AND
BUSINESS
CONTINUITY

Although you cannot plan perfectly for every possible emergency, no one knows your practice better than you. As you move through the planning process, you need to think about maintaining patient and practice continuity as well as business continuity. Planning Checklists and an Office Inventory Checklist are provided in **Appendix D**.

The first document, the **Pre-event Planning Checklist,** consists of a list of broad categories to help you organize your planning activities. Associated with this form is the **Office Inventory Checklist**, an itemized table that will allow you to begin an inventory of your equipment and supplies. Neither is intended to be exhaustive; you need to tailor them to your situation.

In brief, you will need to assess the capacity you already have in each of the following general areas.

Existing plans and policies

- Fire/flood protection plan
- Facility security procedures
- Insurance policies
- Finance and purchasing procedures
- Employee policies
- Risk management plan

> See Appendix D for the Planning Checklists and Office Inventory Checklist, which will facilitate your planning.

Personnel

- Total number of staff types including kinds of skills
- Total number of staff available in an emergency
- Staff potentially vulnerable during an emergency due to limited physical ability, etc.
- Of these, who lives nearby, who lives far away
- Of total staff, number of part-timers

Equipment

- Fire protection and suppression equipment
- Communications equipment
- First aid/triage supplies
- Emergency power equipment
- Personal protective equipment

Backup systems for critical functions

- Offsite storage of paper or electronic medical records
- Payroll
- Communications
- Patient services
- Computer systems

Worried About the Costs of Preparing?

Ready.gov has some ideas on how you can prepare for practice and business continuity that you might not have thought about and includes an estimate of the bottom line for each. A copy of "What Are the Costs?" is also available in **Appendix D**.

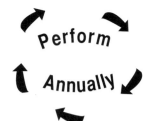
Perform Annually

This part of the toolkit will help you create a plan for your practice. Two clean templates are provided in **Appendix E**, beginning on page 69. Once you have completed the plan, it can be used by you and others in your practice, including those in charge of planning for emergencies and those likely to provide leadership during an emergency. When finalized, office leadership should formally adopt the plan and provide a signed, dated copy to all key staff.

NOTE: There is a national standard—the Incident Command System (ICS)—that will be in use by hospitals, health departments, and others during an emergency and is also used for planning purposes. Office-based practices should become familiar with and use this system, adapting it to their size and circumstances. Additional information regarding the national preparedness efforts, such as the National Incident Management System (NIMS) and the National Response Framework (NRF), are found in **Appendix I**.

Fill in the blanks in the worksheet below to develop the outline of your plan.

Emergency Response Plan

Organization Name: _____

Organization Address: _____

Date: _____

Emergency Response Plan Adopted by:		
Name	**Title**	**Date**

Plan Reviewed and Revised Annually by:

Name	Title	Date

The Practice Emergency Management Team

Staff Name	Home Telephone	Cell Phone	Email

✓ **TIP:** Establish an emergency management team that will be responsible for the development of the practice's emergency response plan. The size of the team will depend on the practice's operations, requirements, and resources. Staff expected to work during an emergency should have pre-approved identification (if available). Check with your local emergency services agency or local health department to determine if there is a standard emergency access ID for health personnel.

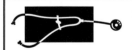 **SMALL PRACTICE TIP:** *The team is the office staff.*

Plan Activation

This plan may be put into action by one of the following individuals (or the person officially designated to fill his/her position during vacation/travel/illness)

Director of the practice site: _____

First backup: _____

Second backup: _____

✓ **TIP:** Activation of practice site emergency response plan may be triggered by:

1. Notification by the local health department that an emergency exists.

2. Notification by a local hospital that an emergency exists.

3. Judgment of the senior decision-maker on-site.

✓ **TIP:** Given limited resources, your practice may well be coordinating with or managed by a hospital or local health department Emergency Operations Center (EOC) during an emergency. But you still need to clarify who is in charge at your physical location to ensure your plan is carried out.

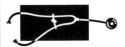 **SMALL PRACTICE TIP:** *Even a small group needs to know how to go into "emergency mode."*

Designate Emergency Operations Center (EOC)

EOC is located at:

✓ **TIP:** Emergency Operations Center (EOC) is a term used in emergency management. For a health care practice, it will be the office where the person in charge is located.

Back-up EOC is located at:

✓ **TIP:** An alternative site is identified in case the main site is inaccessible or too damaged to use.

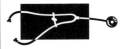 **SMALL PRACTICE TIP:** *The EOC is any place where decisions for your practice can be made—the lead clinician or office manager's office, for example. The space should be big enough to accommodate those who will make key decisions and provide telephone, Internet access, or other back-up communication equipment, if available.*

Communications

Contact List:

Local Professional Society:_____

_____

Banker: _____

_____

Insurance Agent #1:_____

_____

Insurance Agent #2:_____

_____

Staff Contact Information:_____

_____

_____

Critically/Chronically Ill Patients:

_____

_____

_____

Pharmacy:_____

Local EM Coordinator: _____

_____

Local Health Department: _____

Area Hospital: _____

Fire Department: _____

Police Department: _____

✓ **TIP:** Establish methods for how the practice will communicate with local health departments, secondary/affiliated sites, first response units, employees, and patients (on site/off site) about the situation during both operational and non-operational hours. Include back-up methods for communicating with these groups in the event that traditional lines of communication are inoperable.

✓ **TIP:** Communication with your staff, with your patients, and with others in the community is THE KEY to successful emergency response. Be sure to include it in your plan, and consider practicing communication regularly (See STEP 4. INFORM AND PRACTICE, page 27, for details on practicing).

Life Safety/Contingency Planning

Secured Staff Only Areas Include:

1. _____

2. _____

Isolation Areas Include:

1. _____

2. _____

Quarantine Areas Include:

1. _____

2. _____

Waiting Areas Include:

1. _____

2. _____

Assembly Locations:

1. _____

2. _____

Infection Control Measures for Staff, Patients, and Visitors are:

1. _____

2. _____

✓ **TIP:** Identify appropriate methods for protection of assets on site, including staff, patients, equipment, practice site premises, and any vital documentation (patient records, staff contact information, insurance records, etc.).

Establish locations for personnel to assemble in the event that the practice site needs to be evacuated as well as a process for ensuring identification and the safety of all employees during this process. Create a floor plan or map designating these locations.

Develop strategy for site security (i.e., blocking off areas, staff identification) and control of environment (isolation/quarantining measures).

Establish infection control procedures based on practice site criteria for staff and patients.

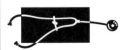

SMALL PRACTICE TIP: *Planning ahead for contingencies (the "what if" list) can be useful. A staff shortage, a supply shortage, and/or other aspects of emergencies may cause contingencies. Alternate use of waiting areas, as well as site/office security, should be considered in developing this section of the plan.*

Contingency Planning SOPs

Staff Shortage:	✓ **TIP:** Plan for operating under sub-optimal conditions. For example, is staff cross-trained to operate machinery, access medical records, and unlock secured areas?
Use of Volunteers:	✓ **TIP:** During an emergency, volunteers may appear at your site, or you may ask for help through your hospital or health department. Do you have a plan for verifying identity and doing a quick orientation for volunteers?
Supply Shortage:	✓ **TIP:** Do you have arrangements with your vendors to deliver supplies if conditions are poor, or do you have arrangements with local vendors or other health care facilities to borrow/share resources?
Space Utilization:	✓ **TIP:** If you are a large facility, you may want to think about how you might accommodate your patients differently than during normal operations. For example, if you to agree to help dispense medications, how would you reorganize your office space to allow patients to flow through easily?
Security:	✓ **TIP:** Consider limiting access into your facility for the purpose of crowd control, or ensure that you have personnel who can assist patients waiting to be seen.

✓ **TIP:** Consider referring to the Event Checklist, pages 57-58, in **Appendix D**, as a tool to keep track of your operations during an event.

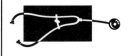

SMALL PRACTICE TIP: *In a small practice, your options may be limited for remaining open. However, if you want to remain open, planning for alternate use of your space is advised and should be a documented part of your plan.*

Roles and Job Action Sheets

The list of roles for staff to assume in an emergency is based on the nationally acknowledged Incident Management System; this ensures consistency across organizations during an emergency. Although individual health care offices are not a mandated part of this system, learning and using these terms will help you coordinate with other parts of the health community, such as the health department or your regional professional society.

Because emergencies can occur at any time and place, it is difficult to assign these roles ahead of time. But it is possible to identify the people most likely to occupy certain roles, such as Incident Commander, Safety Officer, Public Information Officer, etc., during an emergency. Once identified, these staff can be trained and cross-trained, if necessary. A "Job Action Sheet" (JAS) (i.e., assigned roles with specific and predetermined job descriptions) should be developed for each role in advance of an emergency. **Appendix F** (pages 85-97) provides sample JAS that will help you identify specific emergency response roles.

Operations

Roles and Job Action Sheets (JAS):

Incident Commander Potentially Assigned to:

1. _____
2. _____
3. _____

Safety Officer Potentially Assigned to:

1. _____
2. _____
3. _____

Liaison Officer Potentially Assigned to:

1. _____
2. _____
3. _____

Public Information Officer Potentially Assigned to:

1. _____
2. _____
3. _____

Operations Section Chief Potentially Assigned to:

1. _____
2. _____
3. _____

Planning Section Chief Potentially Assigned to:

1. _____
2. _____
3. _____

Logistics Section Chief Potentially Assigned to:

1. _____

2. _____

3. _____

Finance/Admin Section Chief Potentially Assigned to:

1. _____

2. _____

3. _____

Medical/Technical Specialist Potentially Assigned to:

1. _____

2. _____

3. _____

✓ **TIP:** The fact that emergencies can occur at any time and place, these roles cannot be assigned in advance. However, the persons who will most likely occupy each role should be identified so that they can be trained. Remember, any one person may be assigned more than one role.

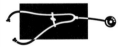 **SMALL PRACTICE TIP:** *If you have a small staff, you may assign more than one function or JAS to a single individual, but you should use emergency preparedness terminology consistently to facilitate coordination with other agencies and local government.*

Because it is recommended that you use standard emergency management language for personnel during an emergency, refer to Appendix F for a list of operational roles for which Job Action Sheets (i.e., assigned roles with specific and predetermined job descriptions) should be developed.

Sample Job Action Sheets (JAS) for each role are also provided.

Demobilization

Notification of Demobilization:

_____

_____

_____

Restocking Supplies and Site Clean-up:

_____

_____

_____

Reimbursement for Services Rendered:

_____

_____

_____

✓ **TIP:** Establish methods for communicating that the situation is over and the practice site will be returning to normal operations. Plan for communication with employees and patients at the health practice site, as well as with any other organizational locations (secondary/affiliated sites), Department of Health, and emergency response agencies.

Establish strategy with suppliers to restock anything used during the emergency.

Establish contact with coordinating agencies about reimbursement for practice site services.

✓ **TIP:** Consider using the Post-event Checklist, pages 59-60, in **Appendix D**, to keep track of your recovery activities and expedite this process.

Incident/Exercise Review and Improvement Plan:

After Action Report Submitted by:

_____

Date:

_____

Improvement Plan Submitted by:

_____

Date:

_____

Changes Needed:

_____

_____

_____

Person Responsible:

_____

Due Date:

_____

✓**TIP:** Recommended to be used for both real emergency or exercise.

Identify those responsible for conducting and writing the after action review for the event.

Assign a time and place to hold the "hot wash" debriefing session shortly after demobilization. Take notes.

Use the debriefing material and any other observations recorded during the incident to create an After Action Report (AAR). This report is a summary of what happened during the event and any lessons identified.

Using the AAR, create an Improvement Plan.

Record changes that are to be made to the plan as well as a timetable for when those changes are to take place, the person(s) responsible for the changes, and when they will be exercised/tested.

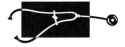

SMALL PRACTICE TIP: _While an emergency event is still fresh in everyone's mind, but after the response is over and recovery is underway, you should review what happened and what needs to be done to strengthen your practice for the next time._

Annual Plan Review

Remember that your emergency plan needs to be updated on an annual basis. For large practices, that includes checking to see if codes and accreditation standards have changed. The emergency preparedness coordinator employed by your local health department or hospital may be able to inform you of key changes in expectations, codes, and standards. If applicable, you (or someone in your practice) should be familiar with the regulations and codes for health care practices as per the following organizations:

- The Joint Commission [formerly known as The Joint Commission on Accreditation of Healthcare Organizations (JCAHO)] standards, if you are JCAHO accredited
- Your specialty's accrediting agency
- Hospital accrediting agencies (if you are so accredited)
- Occupational safety and health regulations
- Environmental regulations
- Fire safety regulations
- Health department codes
- Practice licensing agency standard.

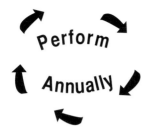

Perform Annually

To improve your chances of maintaining business continuity, once you have an emergency response plan, begin a program of staff orientation and education. Every staff member must know how they will be contacted and what they will be expected to do during an emergency. At a minimum, every staff member needs to learn:

- Family emergency planning (templates are provided in **Appendix A**)
- Likely emergency role(s) and responsibility(ies)
- Notification and communications methods
- Where, when, and to whom to report.

New staff members should receive a basic orientation to the emergency plan on the first day of work. Reinforcement of emergency preparedness can be accomplished with updates at least every quarter, and with a range of emergency drills, and exercises on a regular basis (see "The Exercise Planning Process" below).

Slightly different ongoing training content is needed for three groups of staff—managers, clinical staff, and support staff (those without licenses in one of the health professions)—although the basics of what you expect will be the same. Those in

At-a-Glance: List of Training Resources

- The Centers for Disease Control and Prevention (CDC)

- State and local health departments (contact the Emergency Preparedness Coordinator)

- Federal Emergency Management Agency (FEMA) offers a variety of online courses focused on preparedness

- Hospital(s) with which you are affiliated (contact the Regional Resource Coordinator or EP Coordinator)

- State and local emergency management agencies

- Professional associations to which your agency or staff belong, such as the American Medical Association

management positions (or those who may be assigned to a management role during an emergency) need training on managing others during emergencies and on coordinating with other emergency response organizations in your community. Clinicians need to keep their relevant clinical skills current. Adequately prepared support staff members are critical as they can play a key role in communicating with other staff, patients, and other members of the community and can enable the practice to function effectively.

Emergency preparedness training materials are available from several sources, and a list is provided for you in **Appendix G.**

The Exercise Planning Process

"Exercising" an emergency response plan (i.e., practicing the components of your plan as if an actual emergency were occurring) is essential and can often make the difference between success and failure in an actual crisis. The idea of exercising is not to predict certain events that might happen, but rather to test the ability of the practice to respond to potential emergency events.

Some of the following activities may be beyond the scope of your plan, particularly if you are a small practice and/or it isn't feasible for your practice to participate in community-wide exercises. If that is true for you, see Table 2, Mastering the Basic Steps to Preparedness, for a list of sample exercises that are simple and low-cost ways to exercise the most important aspects of any plan— clear communication and staff preparedness.

Pre-exercise Activities

- Identify exactly what portion of the practice's emergency response will be activated. Use a task list to determine which specific response activities will be practiced.

Example: Set up an Emergency Operations Center (EOC) with complete telecommunications and radio connections between branches and with the county EOC.

- Identify all site personnel who are expected to participate.

- Identify all functional roles (job descriptions) to be activated.

- Prepare observer documents. List evaluation criteria and JAS roles that are to be observed.

Identify the Site Specific Goals and Objectives of the Emergency Exercise

The aim of all exercises is improved preparedness. Clearly stating the overarching goals of the exercise and its specific objectives early on in the planning process increases the likelihood of improvements resulting from the event. The goal of the exercise should clearly state its overall purpose, i.e., "to test our site's collaboration with our affiliated hospital or local health department in response to a tornado." The objectives should state the specific protocols to practice during the event, i.e., "demonstrate how to establish communications with outside organizations" or "how to set up an on-site triage area."

The goals and objectives help everyone involved focus on what aspects of the plan to practice and what actions the staff need to take. Objectives should be challenging but also realistic, achievable, and derived from your practice's emergency management plan. The exercise goals and objectives must also be tailored to the practice's locale and match its emergency plan for it to be an effective assessment and learning tool.

Whether exercising toward a single objective or several, the process should capture the following information for later evaluation:

- the practice's current state of emergency preparedness.

- gaps, weaknesses, or areas of concern affecting the practice's performance as identified through any previous exercises.

- the level of staff knowledge and understanding of emergency preparedness roles and responsibilities.

- the ability of the practice to respond to emerging problems.

Whatever type of exercise you are developing, follow these steps:

- Use practice staff to develop a scenario, which should be based on a possible hazard in your area as determined by your hazard analysis.

- Research and gather background information to make the scenario realistic. For instance, if flooding is a real hazard in your area and you choose that for your scenario, you might want to list the roadways that would likely be closed in order to determine how that might affect staff ability to report to work, as well as patient ability to access medical care, and to test staff knowledge of this potential (and literal) roadblock.

- Draft and review the scenario with the exercise planning team.

- Do a "talk-through" with the entire planning team to identify possible problems and areas that are known to need improvement.

- Finalize the scenario, including the development of simulations and injects (side problems needing solving) required for scenario flow if the exercise includes responding to changing information. For instance, in the flooding scenario, a change might be the water has risen to a higher level and a new street has become impassable, further isolating certain patients and/or disabling communication by telephone.

Exercises should be scheduled as often as possible, with once a quarter being the most common timetable. Even the most routine of events (fire drills, a burst boiler room pipe, etc.) can be used as an opportunity to test the practice's emergency response plan. The exercises are not designed to assign blame but rather to examine the practice's emergency response capabilities. Failures do not necessarily mean that the practice is not prepared; it simply means that some areas of the plan should be re-examined, re-evaluated, and re-tested.

The following checklist is written as if a practice is exercising alone. While this will often be the case, your practice should attempt to participate in at least one community-wide or hospital-associated drill each year.

The exercise planning group (or exercise planner) must:

☐ Secure an appropriate location and supply it with all essential equipment.

☐ Secure space for management of evaluators and observers, providing appropriate communications equipment, orientation materials, identification, and debriefing plans.

☐ Secure space for assembling any "victims," including provision of instructions and transportation to the practice site, if needed.

☐ Prepare signage to direct individuals to assigned locations.

☐ Arrange for equipment specific to the scenario and objectives (e.g., sample collection equipment for an exercise requiring specimens from symptomatic patients; mock medications for a mass prophylaxis exercise).

☐ Secure staff to support the exercise process, including assistance for setup or communications, if needed.

Conduct an Exercise

Conducting an exercise consists of three general steps:

1. Prepare and distribute needed materials and/or equipment; hold briefings.

2. Initiate, facilitate, and observe exercise activity.

3. "Hot wash"/debrief participants.

Standard emergency management procedures require training and exercising to ensure that you are not trying out your plan on the day of the "big flood." See Table 2 for exercise ideas that are simple to execute and test critical aspects of your plan.

Table 2. Master the Basic Steps to Preparedness

Below are a few sample exercises that are simple and low-cost ways to test two of the most important basics of any plan: communication and staff personal preparedness. Remember, exercises do not have to be done on an all or nothing basis. You can start with one office, one floor, one area of your practice; similarly, you can exercise for 15 minutes instead of all day.

Test Communications—Testing your staff phone tree:
At a time when the practice is closed, implement your staff emergency notification procedure, making sure you mention the fact that this is a drill of your emergency response plan. This enables you to assess:

- the accuracy of your staff contact list and
- how long it takes for staff to respond during off hours.

Test Communications—Disseminating information to your patients:
Design risk communication messages and methods to disseminate those messages to your patients concerning their exposure to risk and to determine what makes an effective public response. For example, if the health department announced a possible influenza pandemic and wanted people to stay home and minimize their travel, what message would you put on your voicemail? How would you ensure that the majority of your patients received this message? This exercise will help you:

- Improve leadership comfort by designing new voicemail messages for use during an emergency.

Continued on page 32

Test Communications—Contacting patients during an emergency:
Call patients who are on your "priority patient contact list," that list of patients who will need medical attention within 24 to 72 hours after an emergency. This exercise will help you:

- Keep this list of patients updated and accessible during an emergency;
- Provide patient instructions in the context of what is happening in the community; and
- Test your connectivity to the community emergency response.

Test Personal Preparedness—Assess the status of your staff's personal preparedness plans.
This exercise will help you and your staff to:

- Assess everyone's level of readiness and ability to report to work, if needed, during an emergency;
- Achieve compliance by giving staff time on the job to complete the form, learning from their colleagues how to do so; and
- Assess the likelihood of staff reporting to work during an emergency.

Test Leadership—Develop written and verbal scenarios for leaders or other groups.
This exercise will help you:

- Practice incident commands; and
- Improve decision making.

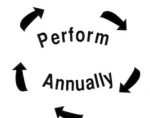

Perform Annually

After any exercise or activation of your emergency plan, you should complete an evaluation to review your response. Changes to the emergency response plan should only be made after such a review has taken place.

Sample Evaluation Questions

Examples of evaluation questions tailored to specific criteria include:

> The Sample Evaluation Questions are available as a blank form in **Appendix H** on pages 101-103.

1. To Evaluate the Practice's Emergency Response Plan:

- Did the plan anticipate all key needs, such as space, communication equipment, and supplies?

- Did the plan include adequate information for communicating with your staff, your patients, and partner organizations?

- Did the plan anticipate all needed jobs or roles?

- Did the plan match the expectations set forth by the surrounding community?

2. To Evaluate What Happened When the Plan Was Put into Actual Use:

- Did the staff go where they were supposed to?

- Did staff follow job (functional role) assignments?

- Was the desired outcome achieved?

3. To Evaluate the Speed with which the Plan Was Put into Place:

- How much time did it take to notify staff of the emergency?

- How much time did it take for staff to take their places?

- How much time did it take to complete other actions that were detailed in the plan?

33

- How did your communication systems function? Were there any problems. If yes, what were they?

4. To Evaluate the Efficiency of Plan Execution:

- Were there repeated messages?

- Any duplicated or conflicting instructions?

- Were supplies wasted?

5. To Evaluate Staff Competency in Specific Functional Roles:

- Were all of the jobs (functional roles) executed? (The functional roles to be assessed must be identified in advance.)

- What was the value of the competency-based training provided to staff prior to the incident? (Competency statements and applicable job action sheets must be incorporated into the assessment.)

Based on answers to the evaluation, observations collected during the exercise, and comments recorded during the "hot wash" debriefing, an After Action Report can be written. This report includes lessons identified during your exercise and notes opportunities for improvement. It is insufficient to say "fix it." Instead, practice leadership should develop an improvement plan that includes:

- a description of actions needed to amend the current plan

- assignments for a particular group or person to create these changes

- an evaluation of the costs and budgetary needs to make the necessary changes

- establishment of a timetable for completing improvements

- a schedule to re-test/re-evaluate the plan once the changes are incorporated.

Suggested Format for an Improvement Plan

Exercise Goal	Evaluation	Needed Change	Person Responsible	Due Date
EXAMPLE 1. Communications: Notify staff of plan activation on weekends	*30% of the phone numbers were out of date*	*Update phone contact information regularly*	*Office Managers*	*July 1 and quarterly thereafter*

The emergency response plan is an ever-evolving document that requires regular evaluation and updating. Failure to do so can result in out-of-date information and procedures that will prevent your practice from functioning during times of crisis.

APPENDICES

Appendix A

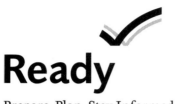

Family Emergency Plan

Make sure your family has a plan in case of an emergency. Before an emergency happens, sit down together and decide how you will get in contact with each other, where you will go and what you will do in an emergency. Keep a copy of this plan in your emergency supply kit or another safe place where you can access it in the event of a disaster.

Out-of-Town Contact Name:_____   Telephone Number:_____

Email:_____

Neighborhood Meeting Place:_____   Telephone Number:_____

Regional Meeting Place:_____   Telephone Number:_____

Evacuation Location:_____   Telephone Number:_____

Fill out the following information for each family member and keep it up todate.

Name:_____Social Security Number:_____

Date of Birth:_____   Important Medical Information:_____

Name:_____Social Security Number:_____

Date of Birth:_____   Important Medical Information:_____

Name:_____Social Security Number:_____

Date of Birth:_____   Important Medical Information:_____

Name:_____Social Security Number:_____

Date of Birth:_____   Important Medical Information:_____

Name:_____Social Security Number:_____

Date of Birth:_____   Important Medical Information:_____

Name:_____Social Security Number:_____

Date of Birth:_____   Important Medical Information:_____

Write down where your family spends the most time: work, school and other places you frequent. Schools, daycare providers, workplaces and apartment buildings should all have site-specific emergency plans that you and your family need to know about.

Work Location One
Address:_____
Phone Number:_____
Evacuation Location:_____

Work Location Two
Address:_____
Phone Number:_____
Evacuation Location:_____

Work Location Three
Address:_____
Phone Number:_____
Evacuation Location:_____

Other places you frequent
Address:_____
Phone Number:_____
Evacuation Location:_____

School Location One
Address:_____
Phone Number:_____
Evacuation Location:_____

School Location Two
Address:_____
Phone Number:_____
Evacuation Location:_____

Work Location Three
Address:_____
Phone Number:_____
Evacuation Location:_____

Other places you frequent
Address:_____
Phone Number:_____
Evacuation Location:_____

Important Information	Name	Telephone Number	Policy Number
Doctor(s):			
Other:			
Pharmacist:			
Medical Insurance:			
Homeowners/Rental Insurance:			
Veterinarian/Kennel (for pets):			

Dial 911 for Emergencies

Ready

Prepare. Plan. Stay Informed.

Family Emergency Plan

Make sure your family has a plan in case of an emergency. Fill out these cards and give one to each member of your family to make sure they know who to call and where to meet in case of an emergency

---

ADDITIONAL IMPORTANT PHONE NUMBERS & INFORMATION

< FOLD
HERE

Family Emergency Plan

EMERGENCY CONTACT NAME:
TELEPHONE:

OUT-OF-TOWN CONTACT NAME:
TELEPHONE:

NEIGHBORHOOD MEETING PLACE:
TELEPHONE:

OTHER IMPORTANT INFORMATION:

Ready

DIAL 911 FOR EMERGENCIES

_____
_____
_____
_____
_____
_____
_____
_____
_____
_____
_____
_____

ADDITIONAL IMPORTANT PHONE NUMBERS & INFORMATION

< FOLD HERE

Family Emergency Plan

EMERGENCY CONTACT NAME: _____
TELEPHONE: _____

OUT-OF-TOWN CONTACT NAME: _____
TELEPHONE: _____

NEIGHBORHOOD MEETING PLACE: _____
TELEPHONE: _____

OTHER IMPORTANT INFORMATION: _____
_____ **Ready**

DIAL 911 FOR EMERGENCIES

_____
_____
_____
_____
_____
_____
_____
_____
_____
_____
_____
_____

ADDITIONAL IMPORTANT PHONE NUMBERS & INFORMATION

< FOLD HERE

Family Emergency Plan

EMERGENCY CONTACT NAME: _____
TELEPHONE: _____

OUT-OF-TOWN CONTACT NAME: _____
TELEPHONE: _____

NEIGHBORHOOD MEETING PLACE: _____
TELEPHONE: _____

OTHER IMPORTANT INFORMATION: _____
_____ **Ready**

DIAL 911 FOR EMERGENCIES

FOLD

FOLD

FOLD

Visit www.redcross.org for more information

Poison Control Center: 1-800-222-1222

Family Doctor :

Ambulance: call 9-1-1 or

Fire Dept.: call 9-1-1 or

Police: call 9-1-1 or

Important Phone Numbers

Emergency Contact Card

American Red Cross

Together, we can save a life

Name:

Home Address:

Household Members Contact Information

Out-of-town contact

Family meeting place outside the neighborhood:

American Red Cross
Emergency Contact Card

Directions:

1. Print this card for each household member.

2. Cut out the card along the dotted lines.

3. Write in the contact information for each household member, such as work, school and cell phone numbers. If you need additional space, use the back side of the card.

4. Fold the card so it fits in your pocket, wallet or purse.

5. Carry your card with you so it is available in the event of a disaster or other emergency when you will want to contact each other.

For more information on creating a family disaster plan and a disaster supplies kit, as well as other valuable disaster preparedness information, visit **www.redcross.org.**

Emergency Preparedness Medical Needs Checklist (for patients)

Dear Patient:

We want you to be ready with your important medical information in case you have to seek medical care in an emergency. Put a completed version of this form in a zip-lock or another waterproof bag and keep it somewhere that is easy to locate. Some people keep it in an envelope on the refrigerator or in their car. Keeping a copy with you and giving a copy to an out-of-town relative will be helpful if you are unable to enter your home.

REMEMBER TO PRINT CLEARLY

Last Name, First Name, Middle: _____

Address: _____

Telephones #: (H)_____(C)_____(W)_____

Primary Care Provider Information

Medical Provider Name: _____

Medical Provider Address: _____

Medical Provider Office Telephone #: _____

Pharmacy Name and Telephone #: _____

Insurance Information

Health Insurance Company: _____

Policy Holder Name: _____

Policy Holder #: _____

Group #: _____

Emergency Contact

Full Name: _____

Telephones #: (H)_____(C)_____(W)_____

Relationship to You: _____

Medical History/Information

I have a history of:

☐ High Blood Pressure   ☐ Seizures   ☐ Infectious Disease: _____

☐ Heart Attack (MI)   ☐ Thyroid   ☐ Psychiatric: type _____

☐ Coronary Artery Disease   ☐ Kidney Disease   ☐ Bleeding or clotting disorder

☐ Stroke   ☐ Diabetes   ☐ Cancer: type _____

☐ High Cholesterol   ☐ COPD   ☐ Asthma

☐ Other_____

_____

_____

_____

_____

_____

_____

_____

_____

*Medication/Rx Information**

Medication/Herbs/Supplements	Dose	Frequency	Reason

*Use attached sheet if you have more medications to list. Do not forget to include over-the-counter medications.

Emergency Preparedness Checklist

I have a seven day supply of essential medications.   YES ☐   NO ☐

I have my important equipment (hearing aid, insulin pump, walker) in a consistent, convenient and secured place.   YES ☐   NO ☐

I have extra supplies (bandages, syringes, infusion set) in an emergency kit.

YES ☐   NO ☐

I have written instructions for anything I will need help with in an emergency.

YES ☐   NO ☐

I have copies of important papers (insurance policies, deeds, stocks, photo ID, passport, social security number, bank account numbers, other financial information, family records—birth, marriage, death certificates).

YES ☐   NO ☐

I have a copy of my medical records with me: YES ☐   NO ☐

Date I obtained copy: _____

Emergency Preparedness Tips

If you have any medical problems or take medications, you should keep a card such as the one on page 48 with you at all times. It covers the following critical items:

☑ **Conditions that a rescuer might need to know about, i.e., diabetes, epilepsy, heart condition, high blood pressure, respiratory condition, etc. (if you are not sure, list it.)**

"My disability, which is due to a head injury, sometimes makes me appear drunk. I'm not!"

"I take Lithium and my blood level needs to be checked every _____ ."

☑ **Allergies and immunizations**

☑ **Medications: If you take medication that cannot be interrupted without serious consequences, make sure this is stated clearly and include:**

Prescriptions (dosage, times taken, administration/regime; i.e., insulin, etc.)

Instructions: i.e., "Take my gamma globulin from the freezer," "Take my insulin from the refrigerator."

☑ **Anticipated assistance needed, for instance:**

"I need specific help with: walking, eating, standing, dressing, transferring."

Walking—"best way to assist is to allow me to hang on your arm for balance."

☑ **Specific communication needs such as:**

"I use a word board, augmentative communication device, artificial larynx, etc., to communicate. In an emergency I can point to words and letters."

"My primary language is (list language here). I am not fluent in English. I will need an interpreter."

☑ **Equipment used such as:**

motorized wheelchair

Instructions: "take my oxygen tank," or "take my wheelchair."

☑ **Sanitary needs such as:**

indwelling catheter

sores

Please visit www.fema.gov for more information on what should be in your disaster preparedness kit.

Sample Emergency Card

To generate an emergency medical card on the Internet, visit
http://www.medids.com/free-id.php.

EMERGENCY MEDICAL CARD

Jane C. Doe   DOB 01/19/1945
225 Main Street
Bethesda, MD 20814

Emergency Contacts:
John Doe (husband)   301-656-7303
Jack Doe (son)   212-442-0995

Physicians:
Primary: R. Smith, MD, 301-656-8800, (c) 646-418-6233
Cardio: A. Jones, MD, 301-699-2300, (c) 646-447-5424

OVER

Conditions:
Heart disease, diabetes

Allergies:
Keflex, peanuts, dairy

Essential Medications:
Dioxin, insulin; taking baby aspirin daily

Assistance needed:
Please bring my insulin from the refrigerator

Equipment:
Syringes on top of refrigerator

Contact Lense Wearer?   ☑Yes   ☐ No

APPENDIX B

How to Become More Involved in Community Emergency Response

- **Health Alert Network**—the Health Alert Network is a connection to the health department; some large urban centers have their own stand-alone system, but most other networks are run by the state department of health. This news system distributes information to users in real time, providing advisories and alerts of important public health and emergency breaking stories.

- **Emergency Services Advanced Registration of Volunteer Professionals (ESAR-VP)**—the system in each state for advanced verification of credentials and licenses of health professionals willing to respond during an emergency event.

- **Medical Reserve Corps (MRC)**—locally organized groups of health professionals and others willing to support the local public health department in an emergency. In some states, entry to the MRC is coordinated with registry in the ESAR-VP system.

- **National Disaster Medical System**—a network of federally organized and supported response groups that train and practice together in order to be ready to set up clinics or hospital services at the site of a disaster.

- **Professional Associations**—your local medical, dental, physician assistant or nursing society may already be engaged with the state health department to provide emergency preparedness resources to its members.

APPENDIX C

Hazard Vulnerability Analysis Form

Practice Name Here: _____

HAZARDS	PROBABILITY	OVERALL IMPACT ON CENTER	OVERALL IMPACT ON COMMUNITY	TOTAL
Natural Hazards				
Flood				
Earthquake				
Tornado				
Hurricane				
Ice/Snow/ Blizzards				
Industrial Hazards				
Fire				
Blackout				
Loss of Water				
Communication Failure				
Gas Failure				
Human-Made Hazards				
Transportation Events/ Incidents				

HAZARDS	PROBABILITY	OVERALL IMPACT ON CENTER	OVERALL IMPACT ON COMMUNITY	TOTAL
Chemical Leaks				
Terrorist Attacks				
Bomb Threats				
Intruder(s)				
Other				
Staff Availability				

Hazard Vulnerability Scale

To calculate your health center's vulnerability to hazards, enter the appropriate number in each box and total for that hazard. We have listed several in each category that are of concern; you may want to add one or more hazards, or describe one of the hazards in more detail, because of your particular local concerns. The higher the point total, the greater the overall impact of the event on the practice site.

"Probability" = the frequency at which the hazardous event occurs.

5 points: Happens annually

4 points: Has happened within the past 2–5 years

3 points: Has happened within the past 5–10 years

2 points: Has happened over 10 years ago

1 point: Has never happened before

"Overall Impact on Center" = the impact that the particular hazard has caused (or could cause) in the way of physical damage to the center, staffing shortages, interruption of patient services, and/or supply disruption.

5 points: Severe impact on center (has caused center to close)

4 points: Significant impact on center

3 points: Moderate impact on center

2 points: Minimal impact on center

1 point: No impact on center

"Overall Impact on Community" = on average, the impact that the particular hazard has caused overall to the wider community in the past.

5 points: Has required a federal response

4 points: Has required a state government response

3 points: Has required a county government response

2 points: Has been resolved with a local response

1 point: No response necessary

You should be certain to include in your plan contingencies for any hazard that scores **10 or higher.** This is not to say that those hazards that fall below 10 points should not be planned for, but rather that greater emphasis should be placed on the more frequently occurring, higher impact hazards.

APPENDIX D

Pre-event Planning Checklist

Organization Name: _____

Organization Address: _____

Name/Title: _____

Instructions: This list is intended to help you remember key components of planning and can be used to track your progress toward a complete emergency plan for your practice. While planning, review this list at least monthly so "In Progress" items are not allowed to wait and are moved to the "Completed" column in a timely manner.

	COMPLETED/DATE	IN PROGRESS	N/A

I. Personnel

	COMPLETED/DATE	IN PROGRESS	N/A
A. Update contact list.	❑ _____	❑	❑
B. Copy of all licenses and hospital privilege documents in a secure place	❑ _____	❑	❑
C. Identify possible assignments.	❑ _____	❑	❑
D. Training plan in place.	❑ _____	❑	❑

II. Equipment

	COMPLETED/DATE	IN PROGRESS	N/A
A. Itemized inventory (photos if needed, check with your insurance carrier).	❑ _____	❑	❑
B. Complete supply list.	❑ _____	❑	❑
C. Backup supplied in an offsite location (if desired).	❑ _____	❑	❑
D. Redundant equipment (if desired/affordable).	❑ _____	❑	❑

III. Space

	COMPLETED/DATE	IN PROGRESS	N/A
A. Emergency activities areas identified.	❑ _____	❑	❑
B. Backup location identified.	❑ _____	❑	❑

COMPLETED/DATE   IN PROGRESS   N/A

IV. Business Continuity

A. List insurance policy numbers, contacts.   ❏ _____ ❏ ❏

B. Backup all business records/licenses.   ❏ _____ ❏ ❏

C. Plan for billing if usual system is not functioning/available.   ❏ _____ ❏ ❏

D. Plan for paying staff if usual system is not functioning/available.   ❏ _____ ❏ ❏

E. Cash reserves and credit plan in place.   ❏ _____ ❏ ❏

V. Patients

A. Emergency information given to all patients.   ❏ _____ ❏ ❏

B. Backup copy of key patient records.   ❏ _____ ❏ ❏

C. List of all most vulnerable patients updated and secured in
offsite location.   ❏ _____ ❏ ❏

D. Remote access to patients' contact and record information.   ❏ _____ ❏ ❏

E. Up to date list of outstanding diagnostic studies.   ❏ _____ ❏ ❏

VI. Communication

A. Emergency plan given to all employees.   ❏ _____ ❏ ❏

B. Backup communication system(s) in place.   ❏ _____ ❏ ❏

Event Checklist

Organization Name: _____

Organization Address: _____

Name/Title: _____

COMPLETED/DATE   IN PROGRESS

If Advance Warning

A. Update vulnerable patient list. ☐ _____ ☐

B. Create a list of outstanding diagnostic studies and consultations to endure followup as soon as possible. ☐ _____ ☐

C. Inform staff of action plan. ☐ _____ ☐

D. Update answering service/Web site information with current emergency information. ☐ _____ ☐

If Evacuated

A. Activate backup communication system. ☐ _____ ☐

B. Coordinate decisions with the hospital, health department emergency management system. ☐ _____ ☐

C. Communicate with staff not on site, as per your plan. ☐ _____ ☐

D. Inform patients, as per your plan, especially most vulnerable patients. ☐ _____ ☐

E. Secure facility. ☐ _____ ☐

F. Secure or evacuate patient and business records, priority given to those patients in diagnostic workup or undergoing complicated medical treatment. ☐ _____ ☐

COMPLETED/DATE   IN PROGRESS

G. Alert financial, insurance, and other agencies as needed.   ❑ _____ ❑

H. Establish temporary record system, if needed.   ❑ _____ ❑

If In-place

A. Activate plan.   ❑ _____ ❑

B. Coordinate decisions with the hospital, health department emergency management system.   ❑ _____ ❑

C. Contact patients on the patient most vulnerable list.   ❑ _____ ❑

D. Update answering service/Web site information with current emergency information as needed.   ❑ _____ ❑

E. Communicate with staff not on site, as per your plan.   ❑ _____ ❑

Post-event Checklist

Organization Name: _____

Organization Address: _____

Name/Title: _____

	COMPLETED/DATE	IN PROGRESS	N/A

I. Personnel

A. Assess personal needs and refer if needed.   ❑ _____   ❑   ❑

B. Obtain new licenses, insurance, privileges information if needed.   ❑ _____   ❑   ❑

II. Equipment

A. Conduct inventory to identify losses and replacements needed.   ❑ _____   ❑   ❑

III. Space

A. Identify damages and needed repairs.   ❑ _____   ❑   ❑

IV. Business Continuity

A. Notify insurance carriers.   ❑ _____   ❑   ❑

B. Work with billing agents and others to re-establish billing mechanism.   ❑ _____   ❑   ❑

C. Retrieve duplicate files to re-establish records.   ❑ _____   ❑   ❑

V. Patients

A. Update answering service/Web site information with current information as needed.   ❑ _____   ❑   ❑

B. Contact most vulnerable patients to re-establish appointment schedule.   ❑ _____   ❑   ❑

COMPLETED/DATE   IN PROGRESS   N/A

C. Identify any gaps in diagnostic testing information and arrange for follow-up or repeat testing.   ❑ _____ ❑ ❑

D. Integrate any emergency or temporary patient records into permanent patient files.   ❑ _____ ❑ ❑

VI. Plan

A. Review all actions and identify needed plan improvements.   ❑ _____ ❑ ❑

Office Inventory Checklist

Organization Name: _____

Organization Address: _____

Name/Title: _____

Instructions: A complete inventory of your office is a good resource for many reasons. This checklist is only a guideline for your needs. Use this template to create a more tailored checklist that reflects your office inventory. Work with your insurance provider to identify the policies that will affect how you would be able to replace items on this list.

	Total number	Value
Business Office		
Desks and chairs		
Side chairs		
Wastebaskets		
Filing cabinets and shelves		
Computers and software		
Printers		
Photocopier		
Dictation machine		
Answering machine		
Bookkeeping equipment		
Fireproof safe for cash and checks		
Secretarial supplies		
Fire extinguisher		
Clocks		
Telephones		
Intercom system		
Doorbell		
Security alarm/video camera		
Batteries		

	Total number	Value
Instruments		
Wall-mounted mercury sphygmomanometers		
Stethoscope(s)		
Wall-mounted otoscope/ophthalmoscope		
Flashlight or light units		
Tongue blades/container		
Reflex hammer		
Tuning forks		
Cerumen remover		
Syringe/plastic bulb		
Disposable vaginal specula/light source		
Disposable sigmoidoscope/light source		
Anoscopes		
Suction set		
Surgical instruments		
Electrocardiogram		
Thermometers		
Cotton-tipped applicators		
Emesis basin		
Glucometer		
Dental instruments (list specific types below)		
Laboratory Equipment		
Microscope		
Centrifuge (hematocrit/urine)		
Hematocrit capillary tubes, sealer		
WBC chambers/pipettes		

	Total number	Value
Sedimentation set		
Incubator		
Urinometer/dipsticks		
Test tubes and racks		
Microscope slides/cover slips		
Bunsen burner/alcohol lamp		
Gram-stain reagents		
10 percent KOH		
Saline		
Refrigerator		
Wax pencils		
Urine culture sets		
Laboratory timer		
Blood drawing equipment		
Strep screen kit		
Stationery		
Letterhead		
Envelopes		
Notepads		
Prescription pads		
Business cards		
Claim forms		
Registration forms		
Consent forms		
School/back-to-work slips		
Laboratory slips		
Appointment calendar		
Reception Room		
Upholstered armchairs		

	Total number	Value
Side tables		
Lamps		
Magazine covers		
Magazines (non-medical)		
Books (non-medical)		
Magazine wall racks		
Plants		
Mirrors		
Paintings		
Children's area		
Television/VCR/stereo system		
Artwork		
Medical literature (pamphlets in various languages specific to area and practice)		
Water cooler		
Printed signs and placards		
Examination Room		
Examination table and stool		
Waiting chairs or sofa		
Eye chart		
Wall cabinet		
Physician's lamp		
Clothes hangers or rack		
Mirror		
Screen or curtains		
Scale		
Artwork		
Weight scale		

	Total number	Value
Dental procedure room		
Standard chair and dental unit		
Compressor		
X-ray machine		
Consultation Room		
Executive desk and chair		
Side chairs (3)		
Bookcase		
Credenza		
Lamps		
Wastebasket		
Dictation machine		
Sharps container		
Biohazards container		
Supplies		
Cloth gowns		
Sheets–paper/fabric		
Assorted syringes/needles		
Assorted tapes		
Assorted gauze pads		
Iodine pads		
Lubricating jelly		
Examination gloves		
Sterile gloves		
Topical skin freeze		
Hemostats		
Soap dispenser		
Bandages		
Alcohol swabs		

	Total number	Value
Patient Comfort Items		
Facial tissues		
Sanitary napkins		
Aspirin/acetaminophen		
Paper cups		
Medication		
Xylocaine		
Oxygen tank		
Morphine		
Diphenhydramine		
Dextrose 50 percent		
IV set-up		
Resuscitation kit		
Dental anesthetics (list names below)		

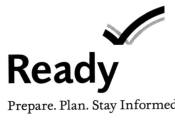

Ready

Prepare. Plan. Stay Informed.

What Are the Costs?

The following will give you an idea of what it may cost to develop a disaster protection and business continuity plan. Some of what is recommended can be done at little or no cost. Use this list to get started and then consider what else can be done to protect your people and prepare your business.

No Cost

- Meet with your insurance provider to review current coverage.
- Create procedures to quickly evacuate and shelter-in-place. Practice the plans.
- Talk to your people about the company's disaster plans. Two-way communication is central before, during and after a disaster.
- Create an emergency contact list, and include employee emergency contact information.
- Create a list of critical business contractors and others you will use in an emergency.
- Know what kinds of emergencies might affect your company both internally and externally.
- Decide in advance what you will do if your building is unusable.
- Create a list of inventory and equipment, including computer hardware, software and peripherals, for insurance purposes.
- Talk to utility service providers about potential alternatives and identify back-up options.
- Promote family and individual preparedness among your co-workers. Include emergency preparedness information during staff meetings, in newsletters, on company intranet, periodic employee emails and other internal communications tools.

Under $500

- Buy a fire extinguisher and smoke alarm.
- Decide which emergency supplies the company can feasibly provide, if any, and talk to your co-workers about what supplies individuals might want to consider keeping in a personal and portable supply kit.
- Set up a telephone call tree, password-protected page on the company website, an email alert or a call-in voice recording to communicate with employees in an emergency.
- Provide first aid and CPR training to key co-workers.
- Use and keep up-to-date computer anti-virus software and firewalls.
- Attach equipment and cabinets to walls or other stable equipment. Place heavy or breakable objects on low shelves.

• Elevate valuable inventory and electric machinery off the floor in case of flooding.
• If applicable, make sure your building's HVAC system is working properly and well maintained.
• Back up your records and critical data. Keep a copy offsite.

More than $500

• Consider additional insurance such as business interruption, flood or earthquake.
• Purchase, install and pre-wire a generator to the building's essential electrical circuits. Provide for other utility alternatives and back-up options.
• Install automatic sprinkler systems, fire hoses and fire-resistant doors and walls.
• Make sure your building meets standards and codes. Consider a professional engineer to evaluate the wind, fire or seismic resistance of your building.
• Consider a security professional to evaluate and/or create your disaster preparedness and business continuity plan.
• Upgrade your building's HVAC system to secure outdoor air intakes and increase filter efficiency.
• Send safety and key emergency response employees to trainings or conferences.
• Provide a large group of employees with first aid and CPR training.

Appendix E

Sample Emergency Response Plan

Organization Name: _____

Organization Address: _____

Date: _____

Emergency Response Plan Adopted by:		
Name	Title	Date
Plan Reviewed and and Revised Annually by:		
Name	Title	Date

The Practice Emergency Management Team:

Staff Name	Home Telephone	Cell Phone	Email

Plan Activation:

This plan may be put into action by one of the following individuals (or the person officially designated to fill his/her position during vacation/travel/illness)

Director of the practice site: _____

First backup: _____

Second backup: _____

Designate Emergency Operations Center (EOC):

EOC is located at:

_____

_____

Backup EOC is located at:

_____

_____

Communications:

Contact List:

Local Professional Society:_____

Banker: _____

Insurance Agent #1:_____

Insurance Agent #2:_____

Staff Contact Information:_____

Critically/Chronically Ill Patients List:_____

Pharmacy:_____

Local EM Coordinator: _____

Local Health Department: _____

Area Hospital: _____

Fire Department: _____

Police Department: _____

Life Safety/Contingency Planning:

Secured Staff Only Areas include:

1. _____
2. _____

Isolation Areas include:

1. _____
2. _____

Quarantine Areas include:

1. _____
2. _____

Waiting Areas include:

1. _____
2. _____

Assembly Locations:

1. _____
2. _____

Infection Control Measures for Staff, Patients, and Visitors are:

1. _____
2. _____

Contingency Planning SOPs:

Staff Shortage:

Use of Volunteers:

Supply Shortage:

Space Utilization:

Security:

Operations:

Roles and Job Action Sheets (JAS):

Incident Commander potentially assigned to:

1. _____
2. _____
3. _____

Safety Officer potentially assigned to:

1. _____
2. _____
3. _____

Liaison Officer potentially assigned to:

1. _____
2. _____
3. _____

Public Information Officer potentially assigned to:

1. _____
2. _____
3. _____

Operations Section Chief potentially assigned to:

1. _____
2. _____
3. _____

Planning Section Chief potentially assigned to:

1. _____
2. _____
3. _____

Operations (cont'd):

Logistics Section Chief potentially assigned to:

1. _____

2. _____

3. _____

Finance/Admin Section Chief potentially assigned to:

1. _____

2. _____

3. _____

Medical/Technical Specialist potentially assigned to:

1. _____

2. _____

3. _____

Demobilization:

Notification of demobilization:

_____

_____

_____

Restocking supplies and site cleanup:

_____

_____

_____

Reimbursement for services rendered:

_____

_____

_____

_____

Incident/Exercise Review and Improvement Plan:

After Action Report submitted by:

_____

Date: _____

_____

Improvement Plan submitted by:

_____

Date: _____

Incident or Exercise Goal	Evaluation	Needed Change	Person Responsible	Due Date
1.				
2.				
3.				

Essential Personnel Call List

1. Administrator: _____

    Phone: (o) _____ (h) _____

    Pager/Cell: _____

    Email: _____

2. Medical Director: _____

    Phone: (o) _____ (h) _____

    Pager/Cell: _____

    Email: _____

3. Center's Disaster Director: _____

    Phone: (o) _____ (h) _____

    Pager/Cell: _____

    Email: _____

4. Security Director: _____

    Phone: (o) _____ (h) _____

    Pager/Cell: _____

    Email: _____

5. Director of Operations: _____

    Phone: (o) _____ (h) _____

    Pager/Cell: _____

    Email: _____

6. Public Information/Media Relations:_____

      Phone: (o) _____ (h) _____

      Pager/Cell: _____

      Email: _____

7. _____:_____

      Phone: (o) _____ (h) _____

      Pager/Cell: _____

      Email: _____

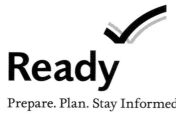

Ready

Prepare. Plan. Stay Informed.

SAMPLE EMERGENCY PLAN

Sample Business Continuity and Disaster Preparedness Plan

☐ **PLAN TO STAY IN BUSINESS**

If this location is not accessible, we will operate from location below:

_____
Business Name

_____
Address

_____
City, State, Zip Code

_____
Telephone Number

_____
Business Name

_____
Address

_____
City, State, Zip Code

_____
Telephone Number

The following person is our primary crisis manager and will serve as the company spokesperson in an emergency.

If the person is unable to manage the crisis, the person below will succeed in management:

_____
Primary Emergency Contact

_____
Telephone Number

_____
Alternative Number

_____
Email

_____
Secondary Emergency Contact

_____
Telephone Number

_____
Alternative Number

_____
Email

☐ **EMERGENCY CONTACT INFORMATION**

Dial 9-1-1 in an Emergency

_____
Non-Emergency Police/Fire

_____
Insurance Provider

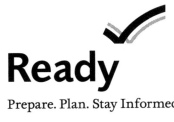

SAMPLE EMERGENCY PLAN

Prepare. Plan. Stay Informed.

Sample Business Continuity and
Disaster Preparedness Plan (cont'd)

☐ BE INFORMED

The following natural and man-made disasters could impact our business.

- _____
- _____
- _____
- _____

☐ EMERGENCY PLANNING TEAM

The following people will participate in emergency planning and crisis management.

- _____
- _____
- _____
- _____
- _____

☐ WE PLAN TO COORDINATE WITH OTHERS

The following people from neighboring businesses and our building management will participate on our emergency planning team.

- _____
- _____
- _____
- _____
- _____

☐ OUR CRITICAL OPERATIONS

The following is a prioritized list of our critical operations, staff and procedures we need to recover from a disaster.

Operation	Staff in Charge	Action Plan
_____	_____	_____
_____	_____	_____
_____	_____	_____
_____	_____	_____

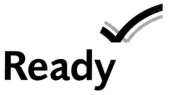

Ready

Prepare. Plan. Stay Informed.

SAMPLE EMERGENCY PLAN

Sample Business Continuity and
Disaster Preparedness Plan (cont'd)

☐ **SUPPLIERS AND CONTRACTORS**

Company Name:_____

Street Address:_____

City:_____ State:_____ Zip Code: _____

Phone:_____ Fax:_____ Email:_____

Contact Name:_____ Account Number:_____

Materials/Service Provided:_____

If this company experiences a disaster, we will obtain supplies/materials from the following:

Company Name:_____

Street Address:_____

City:_____ State:_____ Zip Code: _____

Phone:_____ Fax:_____ Email:_____

Contact Name:_____ Account Number:_____

Materials/Service Provided:_____

If this company experiences a disaster, we will obtain supplies/materials from the following:

Company Name:_____

Street Address:_____

City:_____ State:_____ Zip Code: _____

Phone:_____ Fax:_____ Email:_____

Contact Name:_____ Account Number:_____

Materials/Service Provided:_____

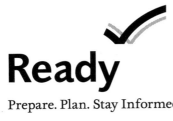

SAMPLE EMERGENCY PLAN

Prepare. Plan. Stay Informed.

Sample Business Continuity and Disaster Preparedness Plan (cont'd)

☐ **EVACUATION PLAN FOR** _____ **LOCATION**

(Insert Address)

- We have developed these plans in collaboration with neighboring businesses and building owners to avoid confusion or gridlock.
- We have located, copied and posted building and site maps.
- Exits are clearly marked.
- We will practice evacuation procedures _____ times a year.

If we must leave the workplace quickly:

_____

_____

1. Warning System:_____

    We will test the warning system and record results _____ times a year.

2. Assembly Site: _____

3. Assembly Site Manager & Alternate:_____

    a. Responsibilities Include:

    _____

    _____

    _____

4. Shut Down Manager & Alternate:_____

    a. Responsibilities Include:

    _____

    _____

    _____

5. _____is responsible for issuing all clear.

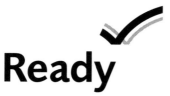

SAMPLE EMERGENCY PLAN

Prepare. Plan. Stay Informed.

Sample Business Continuity and Disaster Preparedness Plan (cont'd)

☐ **SHELTER-IN-PLACE PLAN FOR**_____ **LOCATION**

(Insert Address)

- We have talked to co-workers about which emergency supplies, if any, the company will provide in the shelter location and which supplies individuals might consider keeping in a portable kit personalized for individual needs.
- We will practice shelter procedures _____ times a year.

If we must take shelter quickly:

_____

_____

1. Warning System:_____

      We will test the warning system and record results _____ times a year.

2. Storm Shelter Location: _____

3. "Seal the Room" Shelter Location:_____

4. Shelter Manager & Alternate:_____

      a. Responsibilities Include:

      _____

      _____

      _____

5. Shut Down Manager & Alternate:_____

      a. Responsibilities Include:

      _____

      _____

      _____

6. _____is responsible for issuing all clear.

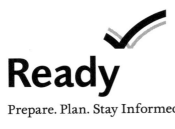

Prepare. Plan. Stay Informed.

SAMPLE EMERGENCY PLAN

Sample Business Continuity and Disaster Preparedness Plan (cont'd)

☐ **COMMUNICATIONS**

We will communicate our emergency plans with co-workers in the following way:

_____

_____

In the event of a disaster we will communicate with employees in the following way:

_____

_____

☐ **CYBER SECURITY**

To protect our computer hardware, we will:

_____

To protect our computer software, we will:

_____

If our computers are destroyed, we will use backup computers at the following location:

_____

☐ **RECORDS BACKUP**

_____is responsible for backing up our critical records including payroll and accounting systems.

Backup records including a copy of this plan, site maps, insurance policies, bank account records, and computer backups are stored onsite_____.

Another set of backup records is stored at the following offsite location: _____
_____.

If our accounting and payroll records are destroyed, we will provide for continuity in the following ways:_____
_____

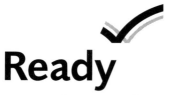

Prepare. Plan. Stay Informed.

SAMPLE EMERGENCY PLAN

Sample Business Continuity and Disaster Preparedness Plan (cont'd)

☐ **EMPLOYEE EMERGENCY CONTACT INFORMATION**

The following is a list of our co-workers and their individual emergency contact information.

_____   _____   _____

_____   _____   _____

_____   _____   _____

_____   _____   _____

☐ **ANNUAL REVIEW**

We will review and update this business continuity and disaster plan in _____

_____.

APPENDIX F

Emergency Management Operational Roles Incident Command Structure

Job Action Sheets

Incident Commander

Safety Officer

Liaison Officer

Public Information Officer

Operations Section Chief

Medical/Technical Specialist

Planning Section Chief

Logistics Section Chief

Finance/Administration Section Chief

Job Action Sheet

Incident Command Structure

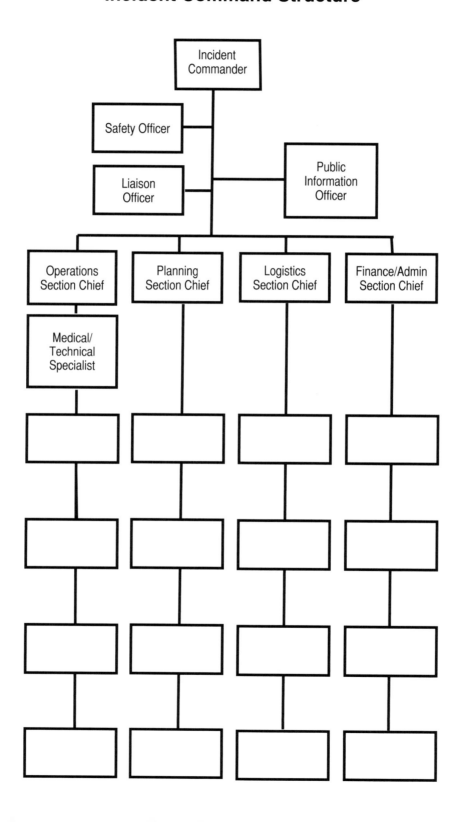

Command Staff   Shift: to _____

INCIDENT COMMANDER

Reports To: Local Chief Health Officer/Hospital Executive

Mission: *Responsible for overall direction of incident management and operations.*

Immediate:

_____ Read this entire JAS.

_____ Establish that an emergency will/has occurred that requires activation of the Emergency Operations Center (EOC).

_____ Activate the EOC.

_____ Command Staff to report to the EOC and are assigned their individual titles [Public Information Officer, Liaison Officer, and Safety & Security Officer (could already be pre-established).]

Intermediate:

_____ Create a Preliminary Incident Action Plan for Command Staff.

_____ Distribute Job Action Sheets to Command Staff (*record the meeting*).

_____ Command Staff identification vests/hats to be put on.

_____ General staff are given their individual titles (Operations Section Chief, Planning Section Chief, Logistics Section Chief, Finance/Administration Section Chief, Medical/Technical Specialist).

Expanded:

_____ Create a preliminary Incident Action Plan for general staff (*record the meeting*).

_____ Distribute Job Action Sheets to general staff.

_____ General staff identification vest/hats to be put on.

_____ Establish schedule for status reports from Command and general staff about operation successes and failures.

_____ Begin operations.

Other Concerns: _____

_____

Command Staff   Shift: to

SAFETY OFFICER

Reports To: Incident Commander

Mission: *Monitors incident operations on all matters relating to operational safety, including the health and safety of emergency responder personnel.*

Immediate:

_____Read this entire JAS.

_____Establish Safety Work Area (this can be your usual desk).

_____Create a Safety & Security Team (if needed).

_____Brief Safety & Security personnel about the emergency at hand, what the plan is, and what is expected from them (*record the meeting*).

_____Distribute Job Action Sheets.

Intermediate:

_____Establish routine briefings with Safety & Security staff.

_____Remove unauthorized persons from restricted areas.

_____Secure the EOC, triage, patient care, morgue and other sensitive/ strategic areas from unauthorized persons.

_____Secure and post non-entry signs around any unsafe areas. Advise Safety & Security staffs to identify and report all hazards and unsafe conditions.

_____Prepare credentialing/screening process of volunteers, patients and their family members.

_____Provide vehicular and pedestrian traffic control, as well as designating waiting areas for victims' families.

_____Secure all food, water, and medical resources.

_____Relay any special information obtained by "specialty" responding personnel to Incident Commander (i.e., information regarding toxic decontamination or any special emergency conditions).

_____Inform Safety & Security staff to document all actions and observations.

Expanded:

____Observe all staff, volunteers and patients for signs of stress and inappropriate behavior. Provide for staff rest periods and relief.

____Communicate frequently with Incident Commander.

Other Concerns: _____

_____

Command Staff   Shift: to

LIAISON OFFICER

Reports To: Incident Commander

Mission: *The point of contact for representatives of other governmental agencies, nongovernmental organizations, and/or private entities.*

Immediate:

_____ Read this entire JAS.

_____ Establish Liaison Work Area (this can be your usual desk).

_____ Create a Liaison Team (if needed).

_____ Contact and brief representatives from outside agencies (Police, Fire, DOH,) that will be responding and/or affected by the incidents about the emergency at hand, what the plan is, and what is expected from them (*record the meeting*).

_____ Distribute Job Action Sheets (if necessary).

_____ Establish routine briefings with outside agencies.

_____ Review county and municipal emergency organizational charts to determine appropriate contacts and message routing.

Intermediate:

_____ Coordinate with Public Information Officer to relay pertinent information to the liaison counterparts of each assisting and cooperating agency (i.e., municipal EOC). Keep them updated on changes and development of Center's response to incident.

_____ Respond to requests and complaints of incident personnel regarding inter-organization problems and needs.

_____ Assist in soliciting physicians and other Center personnel willing to volunteer as Disaster Service Workers outside the Center, when appropriate.

Expanded:

_____ Assure that all communications and inventory of supplies are documented.

_____ Communicate frequently with Emergency Incident Commander.

Other Concerns: _____

Command Staff   Shift: to

PUBLIC INFORMATION OFFICER

Reports To: Incident Commander
Mission: *Responsible for interfacing with the public, media and other agencies with incident-related information requirements.*

Immediate:

_____ Read this entire JAS.

_____ Establish Public Information Work Area (this can be your usual desk) (typically away from the EOC and patient care facilities).

_____ Create a Public Information Team (if needed).

Intermediate:

_____ Work with Incident Commander in crafting a public statement to be released to the media.

_____ Contact and brief representatives from various media outlets about the emergency at hand, what the plan is, what the Center is doing in response, and what information the Center would like to be relayed to the public (*record the meeting*).

_____ Distribute Job Action Sheets (if necessary).

Expanded:

_____ Establish routine briefings with media outlets.

_____ Contact responding agencies' Public Information Officers (PIOs) to coordinate information to be released.

_____ Obtain progress reports from Incident Commander as appropriate.

Other Concerns: _____

_____

_____

Command Staff   Shift: to

OPERATIONS SECTION CHIEF

Reports To: Incident Commander

Mission: *Responsible for managing all tactical operations at an incident.*

Immediate:

_____ Read this entire JAS.

_____ Establish Operations Work Area (this can be your usual desk).

_____ Create an Operations Team.

_____ Brief operations team about the emergency at hand, what the plan is, and what is expected from them (*record the meeting*).

_____ Distribute Job Action Sheets.

Intermediate:

_____ Establish routine briefings with operations staff.

_____ Supervise the execution of all operations mentioned in the Incident Action Plan.

_____ Ensure that adequate communications are being transmitted from the EOC to all operations and vice versa.

_____ Work with Logistics Chief and Planning Chief to ensure that all medical services, ancillary services and human services are being adequately staffed and supplied.

Expanded:

_____ Ensure that all communications, operations and requests are documented.

_____ Communicate frequently with Emergency Incident Commander.

Other Concerns: _____

_____

_____

Command Staff   Shift: to
_____

MEDICAL/TECHNICAL SPECIALIST

Reports To: Operations Section Chief

Mission: *Provides specialty medical advice and assistance to the operations.*

Immediate:

_____ Read this entire JAS.

_____ Establish Medical/Technical Work Area (If necessary, this can be your usual desk).

_____ Create a Medical/Technical Specialist Team (if necessary). Team may include experts in biological/chemical/radiological management, infectious disease control, and pediatric care.

_____ Brief Medical/Technical Specialist team about the emergency at hand, what the plan is and what is expected from them (*record the meeting*).

_____ Distribute Job Action Sheets.

Intermediate:

_____ Establish routine briefings with Medical/Technical Specialist staff (if necessary).

_____ Inventory the number and types of physicians and other specialty staff present.

_____ Coordinate with the Liaison Officer and Security Officer in registering and credentialing volunteer physician/medical staff.

_____ Assist the Incident Commander and Operations Chief in the assignment of medical staff to patient care and treatment areas.

Expanded:

_____ Assist the Operations Chief in developing a medical staff rotation schedule.

_____ Meet with Incident Commander to plan and project patient care needs.

_____ Provide patient priority assessment to Incident Commander to designate patients for early discharge.

Other Concerns: _____

_____

Command Staff   Shift: to
_____

PLANNING SECTION CHIEF

Reports To: Incident Commander
Mission: *Responsible for providing planning services for the incident.*

Immediate:

_____ Read this entire JAS.

_____ Establish Planning Work Area (this can be your usual desk).

_____ Create Planning Team (if needed).

_____ Brief Planning Team about the emergency at hand, what the plan is, and what is expected from them (*record the meeting*).

_____ Distribute Job Action Sheets (if necessary).

Intermediate:

_____ Establish routine briefings with Planning staff (if necessary).

_____ Establish a procedural system ensuring that the collection, formulation, documentation and dissemination of all incident specific data will be handled properly.

Expanded:

_____ Document/update status reports from all section chiefs and inform the Incident Commander on changes occurring to the situation and document/update Incident Action Plan as needed in reference to the changing situation and Incident Commander decisions (do throughout incident).

_____ Communicate frequently with Emergency Incident Commander.

Other Concerns: _____

_____

_____

Command Staff   Shift: to
_____

LOGISTICS SECTION CHIEF

Reports To: Incident Commander
Mission: *Provides all the incident support needs.*

Immediate:

____ Read this entire JAS.

____ Establish Logistics Work Area (this can be your usual desk).

____ Create a Logistics Team: Facilities Unit, Communications Unit, Transportation Unit, Materials & Supplies Unit (could already be pre-established).

____ Brief Logistics Team about the emergency at hand, what the plan is, and what is expected from them (*record the meeting*).

____ Distribute Job Action Sheets.

Intermediate:

____ Designate time for next briefing.

____ Obtain needed supplies with assistance of the Planning Section Chief, Finance Section Chief, and Liaison Officer.

Expanded:

____ Ensure that all communications and inventory of supplies are documented.

____ Communicate frequently with Emergency Incident Commander.

Other Concerns: _____

_____

_____

Command Staff   Shift: to
_____

FINANCE/ADMINISTRATION SECTION CHIEF

Reports To: Incident Commander

Mission: *Responsible for managing all financial aspects of an incident.*

Immediate:

_____ Read this entire JAS.

_____ Establish Finance/Administration Work Area (this can be your usual desk).

_____ Create a Finance Team (if necessary).

_____ Brief finance team about the emergency at hand, what the plan is, and what is expected from them (*record the meeting*).

_____ Distribute Job Action Sheets.

Intermediate:

_____ Establish routine briefings with finance staff (if necessary).

_____ Create an incident financial status report to be submitted as needed to the Incident Commander (typically every eight hours). The report should summarize financial data relative to personnel, supplies and miscellaneous expenses.

Expanded:

_____ Obtain receipts and document ALL expenditures made throughout the incident response.

_____ Communicate frequently with Emergency Incident Commander.

_____ Work with Operations Section Chief on any mutual aid agreements (MOU) and track the financial payouts of the services rendered.

Other Concerns: _____

_____

_____

JOB ACTION SHEET

Position: _____ Person Assigned: _____

Operational Period/Shift: _____ to _____

Reports to: _____

Section/Unit Assigned: _____

Tasks Assigned	**Completed?**

Immediate:

1.	
2.	
3.	
4.	
5.	

Intermediate:

1.	
2.	
3.	
4.	
5.	

Expanded:

1.	
2.	
3.	
4.	
5.	

Other Needs:

_____

_____

_____

_____

_____

_____

Appendix G

Training Material Sources

- The Centers for Disease Control and Prevention (CDC)

- State and local health departments (contact the Emergency Preparedness Coordinator)

- Hospital(s) with which you are affiliated (contact the Regional Resource Coordinator or EP Coordinator)

- State and local emergency management agencies

- Professional associations to which your agency or staff belong, such as the American Medical Association

APPENDIX H

Exercise Flowchart

The exercise process begins with the selection of the type of exercise to be conducted. The flowchart below illustrates this process.

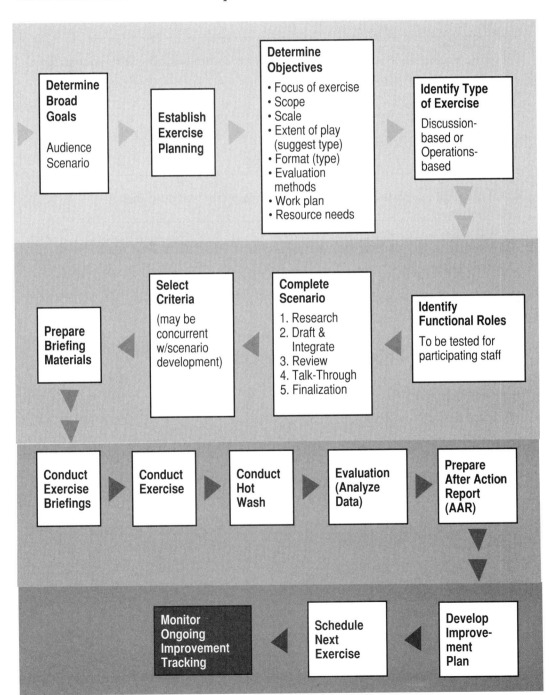

Sample Exercise Evaluation Questions

1. To Evaluate the Emergency Response Plan:

- Did the plan anticipate all key needs, such as space, communication equipment, and supplies?

  _____

- Did the plan include adequate information for communicating with your staff, your patients, and your partner organizations?

  _____

- Did the plan anticipate all needed jobs or roles?

  _____

- Did the plan match the expectations set forth by the surrounding community? _____

2. To Evaluate What Happened When the Plan Was Put into Actual Use:

- Did staff go where they were supposed to?

  _____

- Did staff follow job (functional role) assignments?

  _____

- Was the desired outcome achieved?

  _____

- How did your communication systems function? Were there any problems? If yes, what were they?

  _____

3. To Evaluate the Speed with which the Plan Was Put into Place:

- How much time did it take to notify staff of the emergency?

  _____

- How much time did it take for staff to take their places?

  _____

- How much time did it take to complete other actions that were detailed in the plan?

  _____

4. To Evaluate the Efficiency of Plan Execution:

- Were there repeated messages?

  _____

- Any duplicated or conflicting instructions?

  _____

- Were supplies wasted?

  _____

5. To Evaluate Staff Competency in Specific Functional Roles:

- Were all of the jobs (functional roles) executed? (The functional roles to be assessed must be identified in advance.)

  _____

- What was the value of the competency-based training provided to staff prior to the incident? (Competency statements and applicable job action sheets must be incorporated into the assessment.

  _____

APPENDIX I

Resources

American Red Cross

http://www.redcross.org/ (external link)

Federal Emergency Management Agency (FEMA)

http://www.fema.gov/ (external link)

Ready America

http://www.ready.gov (external link)

Ready New York for Businesses

http://nyc.gov/html/oem/downloads/pdf/Business_Guide_Final.pdf

Ready New York Household Guide

http://www.nyc.gov/html/oem/downloads/pdf/household_guide.pdf

World Health Organization

http://www.who.int/en/ (external link)

codeReady Minnesota

www.CodeReady.com

Lyznicki J, Subbarao I, Benjamin G, James J. Developing a Consensus Framework for an Effective and Efficient Disaster Response Health System: A National Call to Action. *Disaster Medicine and Public Health Preparedness - 1(Supplement_1): 51-54 2007*. © 2007 American Medical Association and Lippincott Williams & Wilkins. DOI: 10.1097/DMP.0b013e31814622e2

The New York Consortium for Emergency Preparedness Continuing Education (NYCEPCE) offers training materials and courses that can be used in your preparedness activities. These can be found on our Web site at:

Online courses: **http://nycepce.org/CourseList.htm**
In Person Training: **http://nycepce.org/news.htm**
Training Materials: **http://nycepce.org/resources.htm**

INDEX

Numbers in italics refer to figures and tables.

NOTES

NOTES

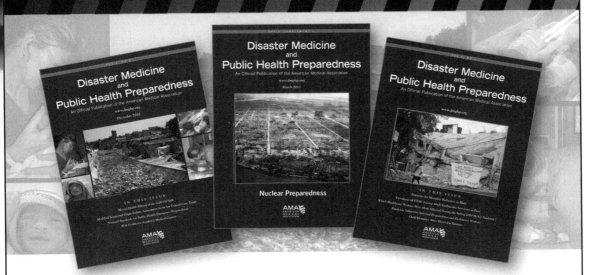
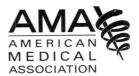

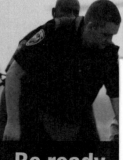
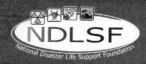